THE
MEETING

THE
MEETING

For the Families & Friends of Alcoholics

Lois Barleycorn Dickens

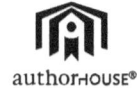

authorHOUSE®

AuthorHouse™
1663 Liberty Drive
Bloomington, IN 47403
www.authorhouse.com
Phone: 1-800-839-8640

Published by AuthorHouse   03/24/2012

ISBN: 978-1-4678-9633-7 (sc)
ISBN: 978-1-4678-9634-4 (e)

Any people depicted in stock imagery provided by Thinkstock are models, and such images are being used for illustrative purposes only.
Certain stock imagery © Thinkstock.

This book is printed on acid-free paper.

Because of the dynamic nature of the Internet, any web addresses or links contained in this book may have changed since publication and may no longer be valid. The views expressed in this work are solely those of the author and do not necessarily reflect the views of the publisher, and the publisher hereby disclaims any responsibility for them.

For the Loved Ones of Alcoholics

To A & H—they know who they are.

The Meetings

Meeting 1

Tonight's Topic—Why do I keep coming back?

AL stands for Alcoholics' Loved Ones and is a meeting for anyone who is, or has been, affected by someone else's drinking, regardless of whether the person is still drinking or not.

MACK says,

"Ok, shall we make a start?

One of the disciplines in AL is that we start on time and we finish on time, regardless.

So, I will read the suggested opening:

We would like to welcome you to this AL meeting.

The AL meeting is a group of relatives and friends of problem drinkers who share their experience, strength and hope in order to solve their common problems. We believe alcoholism is a family illness and that changed attitudes can aid recovery.

For the benefit of our two newcomers, Josh and Ingrid, who are here tonight I would like us to go round the room and introduce ourselves, using first names only and if anyone chooses to, they can say who the problem drinker is in their lives."

Meet the Group

MACK

"So I will start with myself. I'm Mack and I am chairing the meeting tonight. The person in my life who has a drink problem is my son."

CLARISSA

"Hello, I'm Clarissa and the alcoholic in my life is my husband. He was in Alcoholics Anonymous (AA) for 2 years but he recently picked up again and is currently off the wagon. I'm hoping he decides to go back to AA but I know that has to be his decision, I cannot force him to go. I am here tonight for me."

ELSA

"Hello, my name is Elsa and I am an adult child of an alcoholic (ACOA). The alcoholic in my life is my father."

JEFF

"My name is Jeff and the person with the drink problem in my life is my son. He is still drinking heavily and is drunk most days. He shows no interest in seeking help for himself but I need to come here to get help for me so I can cope with having him in my life."

ALICE

"Hello, I'm Alice and I'm married to Jeff. We come along to the meeting together because, as he said, it's our son who has a problem with alcohol."

VICKY

"Hello, my name is Vicky and the problem drinker in my life is my daughter."

FADIA

"Hello I'm Fadia and the person whose drinking I have been affected by was my grandfather. I was sent to live with my grandparents when I was young and found myself caught up in the chaos caused by his drinking."

KALEB

"Hello, I'm Kaleb the drinker in my life is my wife. I haven't been coming here long. My wife hasn't had a drink for 3 months but she's 'white knuckling' it. Because she is trying to stop drinking herself, without any support, I fear for her picking it up again. I feel as if I'm always living on a knife edge. Every time I get home from work and put my key in the lock I never know what I'm going find on the other side of the door."

EDDIE

"Well I'm Eddie and as most of you know I'm a 'double-winner'. For the newcomers here that simply means I'm a member of two support groups. I'm a recovering alcoholic so I'm in AA but I'm also married to a recovering alcoholic so I qualify for membership of AL too."

JOSH

"Hello, my name's Josh and I am a medical student. The drinker in my life was my twin sister. She died last year."

He pauses to compose himself.

"I have never been to an AL meeting before so I don't really know what to expect. My counsellor told me about the group and suggested I come along."

STAVROS

"Hello, I'm Stavros and the person with the alcohol problem was my wife. Whether she is still alive or not, I don't know. The last time I heard any news of her, she was spotted living on the streets in Sheffield but I have never been able to track her down."

INGRID

"This is my first meeting ever. It's my husband who drinks too much and he is ruining my life. I am on anti-depressants and I think I am going to have a nervous breakdown if he doesn't stop soon . . ."

Ingrid begins to sob uncontrollably and wipes her eyes. Shaking her head she indicates that she cannot say anything else at present.

Mack reassures Ingrid.

Mack is chairing the meeting tonight and he is a regular at AL meetings. He is a man of around 60 and comes from a family of Irish descent. He retired on grounds of ill-health at 52, which he believes is the result of obsessively trying to stop his alcoholic son from drinking.

MACK

"Don't worry Ingrid we all do that when we first come in. If you just sit and listen to others in the group tonight then hopefully you will be able to take something away with you that will give you some comfort in your current situation and will make you want to come back and get more of what's on offer here.

Also I should point out that this is an anonymous group and that no one gives their surnames. We don't even have to give our real first names if we don't want to. Anonymity is one of the key principles we adhere to in the group.

You do not need to tell us who you are, where you live, where you work, what you do—absolutely nothing about your personal details at all if you don't want to.

Most of us will not be telling you about ourselves. There are 12 of us here tonight but the numbers vary every week and sometimes there are more and sometimes less. People come and go as they please. Some stay some don't.

4

You don't have to come every week but we do suggest you attend as regularly as you possibly can if you want to benefit from what's on offer. Our only reason for being here is to share our experience, strength and hope to help ourselves and each other to gain some peace of mind because our lives have been impacted on by somebody with an alcohol problem.

Anything else about your life is no concern of ours unless you choose to share it with us. If you don't want to share personal information, nobody will ask you about it or think any less of you in any way.

And so, on with the meeting, as I've said my name is Mack and although I am chairing the meeting tonight, I'm only doing it for this month. In AL we have rotation of leadership so no one is in charge. We rotate any work that needs to be done. So this month it's me but next month it will be someone else who volunteers to Chair.

A special word for the newcomers, it may all seem very strange at first and you will probably go away not understanding much about what you hear tonight. But if you feel something that brings you back then that is enough to be going on with. Just keep coming back and it will eventually all start to become much clearer about what support you can get here.

Also, although we meet up in a church hall this programme is not religious and has no connection to any church. The only reason we meet here is because of low costs.

So on with the meeting. Every week we have a different theme and tonight's theme is:

Why do I keep coming back to AL?

Clarissa can you start us off with the 12 steps please?"

CLARISSA

"**Step 1:** We admitted we were powerless over the problem drinker and that our lives had become unmanageable."

ELSA

"**Step 2:** We came to believe that a power greater than ourselves could restore us to serenity."

JEFF

"**Step 3:** We made a decision to turn our will and our lives over to the care of our higher power (HP)."

ALICE

"**Step 4**: We made a searching and fearless moral inventory of ourselves."

VICKY

"**Step 5:** We admitted to our HP, to ourselves and to another human being the exact nature of our wrongs."

FADIA

"**Step 6**: We were entirely ready to have our HP remove all these defects of character."

KALEB

"**Step 7**: We humbly asked our HP to remove our shortcomings."

EDDIE

"**Step 8**: We made a list of all persons we had harmed and became willing to make amends to them all."

JOSH

"**Step 9:** We made direct amends to such people wherever possible, except when to do so would injure them or others."

STAVROS

"Pass."

INGRID

"**Step 10:** We continued to take personal inventory and when we were wrong promptly admitted it."

MACK

"**Step 11:** We sought through reflection and meditation to improve our conscious contact with our HP, seeking only knowledge of our HP's will for us and the power to carry that out."

CLARISSA

"**Step 12**: Having had an emotional and spiritual awakening as the result of these Steps, we tried to carry this message to others, and to practice these principles in all our affairs."

MACK

"I've asked Elsa to be our main sharer for tonight and can I just remind you that there is no obligation for anyone to share. You can remain silent and just listen if you wish but those who do decide to share are allowed to do so without interruption from others.

So over to you, Elsa on the theme of:

Why you keep coming back?"

Elsa is a long time member and has progressed through the early stages of recovery. She can now speak about her experiences with an air of confidence and emotional detachment which the newer members are unable to do.

<u>ELSA</u>

"One of the first things I always like to start my shares with is to thank everybody for being here tonight because without you all I wouldn't have a meeting to come to.

What I like about coming here is that it is not just a drink-o-log. We don't sit around focusing on the drinker and highlighting all of their diary events of the past week. We actually get to talk about the programme and we get to focus on ourselves and our own recovery from the impact the drinker has had on our lives.

I come to AL because I need to hear other people's perceptions about this programme. I need to hear newcomers say what they don't understand and I need to hear those who have been around for a long time to say what they do understand and have learned and experienced.

I think the basic principle of AL is that we help and support each other. Whenever I come to a meeting I go away feeling stronger. I think when you reach your rock bottom you will reach out for anything and that's exactly how it was with me when I first came in here. Growing up with a drinking parent had distorted my thinking and feelings to such an extent that I didn't know which way was up and which way was down. I had to take it very gently at first. The Steps were just a blur to me I couldn't make head nor tail of them. It just sounded all double-dutch to me. So what I started with was the slogans on the table."

Elsa points to numerous cards propped up along the middle of the table with various slogans written on. 'Keep it Simple'. 'Easy Does

It'. 'Listen and Learn'. 'Live and Let Live'. 'First things First'. 'One Day at a Time'. 'Think' and so on . . .

"My favourite slogan was *'Easy Does It'*. It allowed me not to expect too much of myself. It helped enormously being able to just sit quietly week after week and listen to more experienced members and learning what they had tried in their situations that had worked for them. I was told to take what I liked and leave the rest. That's exactly what I did. Most of it I couldn't understand anyway but even though I didn't understand it at the time it had still registered in my mind. It's amazing how much of that stuff came in useful later on down the road when it all started to make sense. The fog slowly began to lift and I was able to take more on board. I now get my answers from the shares that people give in this room. Someone will say something and suddenly my ears prick up and I can identify something which had previously been hidden from myself under layers of denial.

I know it isn't until I'm aware of something that I can ever have any hope of looking at it and seeing more options. Today I have choices because of AL. I am now much more aware of myself and as such have a greater understanding of where my own strengths and weaknesses lie. I can make better choices for myself because today I know what suits me and what doesn't. AL has taught me the principle of taking my hands off the drinker and focusing on my own life.

Well, I don't want to go on and on because I'm aware that there are 12 of us here and if everyone is going to have the opportunity to share I won't take up any more of the group's time tonight.

I will just leave it there Mack."

MACK

"Thanks Elsa. So that just leaves me to throw open the meeting for anyone who wants to come in and share."

There is silence for approximately 25 seconds and everyone around the table looks deep in thought. Mack sits patiently; he does not try to encourage anyone to speak.

FADIA

"May I come in Mack?"

Fadia has been in the group for some time and like Elsa can speak in a way which reveals her years of experience of sharing her feelings.

"I would like to thank Elsa for her share I got a lot of identification out of that. On the point of AL being for us and not the drinker I would like to share parts of my experience around that. About 5 years ago I went for 6 counselling sessions organised by my doctor. My nerves were so bad he referred me to a therapist. I told her I had just recently joined AL and that I found it very helpful.

I thought she had understood me. However, after the 6th session was almost over she said she thought I was doing very well to say I was an alcoholic! I couldn't believe my ears. How could she have got it so wrong. I was furious. I felt so let down, I felt a sense of failure really. When I had said I go to a group for the loved ones of alcoholics she had only heard the alcoholic bit and had just jumped to the conclusion that I was an alcoholic!

So the whole of her counselling over the previous 6 sessions just flew out of the window for me. I thought how well could she have been listening to me if she had got that so wrong? She hadn't bothered to check it out or discuss it in more detail over the whole time I'd spent with her. How annoying it felt to experience that from someone I was led to believe was qualified to help me. But what the experience did do for me was it gave me a comparison. I could look at her help and compare that with the help I get here in AL, where I can just come in and be accepted immediately without having to go into great explanations about myself and that to me, is priceless, so that's why I keep coming back."

GROUP TOGETHER

"Thanks Fadia".

Vicky gestures with her hand and starts to speak.

Vicky is a relatively recent member of AL but she has spent a couple of years chaperoning her daughter to AA meetings. She is desperate to gain as much knowledge from others as she can in as short a space of time as possible, she feels angry that this problem is taking up so much of her life.

VICKY

"Thank you everybody for being here.

So, Why do I keep coming back?

Where should I start?"

She sighs.

"I suppose I need to start with an apology. I need to apologise to everyone in AL because I went to AA for years. I didn't want AL. I wanted to fix my daughter's drinking problem myself and no one but no one was going to stop me! I wanted to conquer alcoholism single-handedly and I knew best.

Over the years many people in AA took me to one side and quietly suggested that I find help for myself. Some people suggested AL to me but I just continued to ignore everybody. As I said I knew best. In my mind my daughter was my responsibility and I'd managed to fix everything else in her life up until now so I couldn't see that this problem should be any different.

I frog-marched my daughter to AA and sat in meetings with her for nearly 2 years just to make sure she didn't leave halfway through. I was totally obsessed with her drinking. Meanwhile I had stopped living my own life and put it on hold. My daughter had become my whole life even though she was nearly 26 years old.

But with all my efforts and obsessive vigilance of her, what did she do? Yep, she started drinking again and ended up on a life-support machine needing a liver transplant. She died twice in the hospital and had to be resuscitated. It was only then that I hit my rock bottom and thought I can't do this anymore. I felt totally beaten. It was then that I finally threw in the towel and swallowed any shred of pride I had left and crawled into AL. It was incredible pain that brought me here.

That was 10 months ago and today I do fully accept I need to be in this group. I am so grateful to be here tonight and to feel as emotionally strong as I do. It is a slow process for me but one day at a time I feel I am getting on top of this because I have learned some great tools in here for dealing with it.

I have learned about detachment. I had no idea how to detach before I came in here. I'd never been able to step-back and let my daughter make her own choices. I wanted her to do what I wanted. Now the spirituality of the programme for me is having peace and serenity in my own life. Learning from everyone else's experience, strength and hope has given me the ability to end my struggle and stop trying to control my daughter, it's her problem not mine and she has to deal with it in her own way.

Today I respect AL and what it has to offer me. I don't want to sit in AA meetings anymore getting involved in my daughter's business. I'm glad we don't have AA literature on our table and I don't want this to be an AA meeting because I don't get my identification from AA people. I get more for me personally out of listening to AL members. I now like to be with people who are suffering with the effects of someone else's drinking. I love this safe haven and I want that healing that I get in here.

I would find it too much for me to sit in an AA meeting now because I know there is a part of me that doesn't 'Keep my hands off'. I want to get in there and sort them all out. Years ago I tried everything, I tried drinking with the alcoholic, I tried not drinking with her. I think I had a belief that I could somehow take away her pain and I couldn't and me trying to do that just ended up all going sour on me.

Nothing I did ever worked but that didn't stop me from trying every mortal thing under the sun week in and week out. They say the definition of insanity is to keep doing the same things over and over again and expect to get different results—well by that definition I was well and truly nuts. I kept wading in there and ignored all my failures. It was only at my first meeting, which just happened to be about Step 1, that I heard people sharing about their experiences of trying to control the drinker and how futile they had found their efforts to be.

After the meeting that night I felt as if a huge weight had been lifted off my shoulders. Once I accepted that I could not change the drinker's behaviour I was finally able to give myself permission to stop trying. My acceptance freed me from my compulsion to control my daughter's drinking and I felt a shift in my perspective. I felt lighter than I had done for years. I still feel lighter when I leave these meetings and that's why I keep coming back.

And I'll just leave it at that Mack."

GROUP TOGETHER

"Thanks Vicky."

Another short silence then Eddie motions to come in.

Eddie is an alcoholic and has been a member of AA for 20 years. He has been sober for 18 years. He is a semi-retired university lecturer. He joined AL 18 months ago.

<u>EDDIE</u>

"Thank you everybody for being here.

So, why am I here tonight?

A quip I once heard in AA was that 'I'm here because I'm not all there'."

Everybody laughs.

"Well, that seems to fit the bill for me.

As most of you know I am a double-winner! For the newcomers, this basically means I am in both support groups. I'm a member of AA and also I'm a member of AL. I can see you are looking puzzled. Yes, I am a recovering alcoholic but I haven't had a drink for 18 years, however, I still accept that I have the illness of alcoholism but I manage to keep it in remission, so to speak, by working the AA's 12 Step Programme to discipline my behaviour so that I do not have the compulsion to drink anymore.

So why am I here? Well, because I am married to Sarah who is a recovering alcoholic too, so that makes me qualify to be in this group as the loved one of an alcoholic. You might think that after 20 years in AA I would know the 12 Step Programme like the back of my hand—and I do—but we are looking from a different vantage point in AA than we are in AL. In AA it's all about me keeping sober. In AL it's mainly about my relationships with other people. So I find this is a completely new way of using the programme from what I am used to.

I have been coming along to AL now for 18 months and my wife thoroughly recommends it. She tells everybody in AA that I am so much better to live with than I have ever been. I can honestly say she is now a great advocate for AL because she has seen the rewards to be gained from it.

By the way you would be amazed to realise how many people out there . . ."

He gestures towards the door.

". . . believe that AL is somehow part of AA. Part of the same organisation. We are not part of AA. The two groups are totally separate.

A lot of people think that just because we also use a 12 Step programme we must be attached in some way. Believe me AA has enough problems of their own to deal with without joining itself at the hip to AL or any other drink treatment association for that matter! Both AA and AL stand alone. I think it is important for us to try and get that message across to people because I think it may be causing confusion and stopping some people from coming along for the help and support they can get from us. Anyway, enough of my soap-box and back to why I keep coming back.

I keep coming back because when I come here there is sanity in this room. For me the group is my guide, my HP, so to speak. I find twelve heads are better than one when I am trying to solve my problems. I find coming to meetings is a small price to pay for what I get back in peace of mind. I can come here and realise that some of my significant others have major issues in their lives but that they have got to sort them out for themselves, it is not my job to take over their lives for them. They are not my issues.

I find there is always someone here who is on a higher vantage point to myself so I can find out what's down the road for me. I used to live my life thinking if only she stopped behaving badly my life would be a bed of roses but now I know it's not that simple. I have played a part in this drama too. I have picked up other people's responsibilities. I have made excuses for others bad behaviour. I have been guilty of not taking sufficient care of myself and my own life. I have not honestly expressed my feelings and thoughts.

In AL I am learning to own up to my part in things and to identify where my true responsibilities lie and make a commitment to taking care of myself and my own matters.

In here I feel I have been loved back to health. On the night's I can't make the meeting perhaps because I am thousands of miles away on business, at 7.30 on a Monday evening, I will think to myself well they will just be going into the meeting now and I miss you all.

I feel the power of meetings is marvellous. I come out a different person because I am able to mix with others who understand, who have been there themselves and know without having to be told where I am coming from."

At this point Ingrid interrupts Eddie's share.

INGRID

"But are you all saying there is nothing we can do to stop the drinker from drinking?"

Because Ingrid is a newcomer and doesn't realise that the format of the meeting is to allow others to share without being interrupted, she has stopped Eddie in his tracks. Mack is aware that in his role as Chairperson he should stop Ingrid and suggest she wait until Eddie has finished his share, however, he uses his discretion and allows the cross-talk. Eddie realises what Mack is doing and happily lets Mack respond to Ingrid's question.

MACK

"Well yes, it's true we cannot control the drinker, in that, if they want to get alcohol no matter what we try to do to stop them they will find it anyway. Even if we stand guard over them 24 hours a day you would be amazed at the tricks they will get up to if they want to find a drink.

A lot of people come in here looking for a magic pill to take home with them to feed to the drinker which will magically stop them from drinking any more. If such a pill existed we could all go home now and the problem would be history. As it is—there is no magic pill. However, that doesn't mean we are helpless in the situation.

What our experience has shown us is if we change our behaviour by coming to meetings and learn a different way of being in the drama then very often the alcoholic develops a desire in themselves to change too. So we change first and they very often, not always, but very often the drinker changes their patterns too. They haven't much choice really because if we are no longer performing the same role as we have always done then the drinker is left without a dance partner, so to speak. That might all sound very complicated for your first meeting and it is but I can only suggest that you keep coming back and *'Listen and Learn'*, which is another one of our slogans.

We can have a great influence on the alcoholic but not in the way that we had all thought before coming into this room. Our experience has shown us that often the best way to deal with an alcoholic is to be counter-intuitive. To do the very opposite to what we ourselves feel would help! I have found that myself with my alcoholic son. I have no idea why it works I only know it does.

Maybe a top psychiatrist could tell us all why it works - but it's enough for me to know it does work. So I practice it in my life and so far I have got far better results than I ever got trying to use only my own head to solve the problem. The alcoholic was running rings around me and I was chasing after him like a headless chicken but nothing ever changed.

Once I *'Let Go'* of him he found AA himself and has been sober, on and off, now for 3 years. His drink problem is now his problem, not mine and so far he seems to be picking up the responsibility for it much more so than he ever did when I was constantly circling around him.

Just keep coming back Ingrid and Josh and keep asking questions both before and after the meeting. You can also choose a sponsor from the group if you feel you need support between meetings or you feel you have anything to share but feel it is too personal to share with the whole group.

So Eddie, would you like to come in again and finish your share?"

EDDIE

"Thanks Mack. I would just like to come in on your last point Mack about curing the alcoholic. Speaking as a recovering alcoholic myself I can share with Ingrid my own experience of giving up the booze. I haven't had an alcoholic drink for 18 years.

I can tell you all that before I made the decision myself nothing anyone could have said would have made me stop drinking. I knew my mother would always pick me up, brush me down and I could start all over again. She made it easier for me to drink. In my case it was only when my mother was no longer there to pick me up that I was forced into taking responsibility for my own excessive drinking habits.

Once I got into AA and got sober my brain was freed up to start sorting out my condition. I now firmly believe it is not the drinking, it's the thinking, which is the core problem with an alcoholic. Well with this alcoholic anyway. I was always floundering because of my faulty or maybe just different thinking patterns. I never wanted to take responsibility for my life. I wanted someone else to do everything for me. Whenever life got too tough for me I would just look to someone else to fix-it for me.

I would manipulate everyone around me to make my life easier. My first wife got sucked into the parent role with me so I ended up behaving more like her naughty teenage son rather than her husband. It was none the wonder that she felt as if she was going around the bend! My behaviour forced her into the parent role with me.

My advice to any loved one of an alcoholic. Sorry not my advice we do not give advice in AL we only make suggestions based on our own experience. So a suggestion I would make to the loved ones of an alcoholic based on my own experience would be to *'Look after Yourselves First'* and emotionally detach from the alcoholic because they will, I know I certainly did, use any emotional attachment you have towards them to manipulate you into propping them up. My mother and then my wife were emotionally manipulated into looking after me as if I was a child not an adult man.

I learned in AA that I can't just sit around waiting for something to happen. I had to learn to make things happen myself. I had to learn to initiate and stop waiting for someone else to sort my life out for me. The 12 Step Programme in AA changed my life, it overrides my own naturally distorted thinking and allows me to manage my life better than I have ever been able to before. Now I have also found AL I am learning how better to deal with my relationships with others.

All I know is my relationships are better today and that is testimony to the 11 people sitting in this room tonight and that's why I keep coming back."

GROUP TOGETHER

"Thanks Eddie."

CLARISSA

"Can I come in Mack?"

Clarissa is women in her mid 30's with 3 young children and an alcoholic husband who is in AA. She is often very emotional in meetings.

"Well I'm pleased to be here even though I haven't been for a while. And welcome to the newcomers I know how difficult it is to walk through those doors for the very first time. You have both overcome a huge hurdle by having the courage to get yourselves here and I do hope you get something out of it.

The alcoholic in my life is my husband. I shouldn't really call him an alcoholic, that is for him to say but it's enough to say I'm here because my life was being badly affected by his excessive drinking.

Before I came into AL I think I just felt it was my duty to stay in the marriage and put up with his unacceptable behaviour. I was doing everything to suit him. I got myself so exhausted. I was incredibly resentful that I seemed to be the only one stepping forward to try and sort him out. The rest of my family just washed their hands of him and told me to leave him. But I didn't want to leave him and I didn't want to divorce him. But I was so far down I was crackers. I wanted a bus to come and get me. I wasn't suicidal, I couldn't have done it myself but I did wish that a bus would mount the pavement and end it all for me. When he threatened to take an overdose and top himself I told him to do me a favour and get on with it! That's how bitter and twisted my thinking had become because of the effects his drinking had had on me.

However, in AL I've learned that events are not necessarily the problem. The problem can often be my reaction to events. Of course my husband does have the power to affect my feelings but I also have the power to decide how much of his baggage I am going to allow into my thinking. I can decide I am not letting his chaotic behaviour derail me. I can decide that I am not going to allow myself to be pushed into accepting his responsibilities.

Now I am trying to 'wear life like a loose garment'—as they say in AL."

Clarissa stops speaking as she struggles to control her feelings. She wipes a tear away and continues.

"I am trying not to be so much of a reactor to my husband's antics. The slogan 'Think' helps me a lot in trying to step back and give myself thinking time before I jump in to the fray.

He didn't half lead me a merry dance when he was drinking did he not? When I first came in here I was not ready to listen. I was too hurt and emotionally vulnerable for that. I had to be allowed to indulge in just letting off steam week after week. I had to be able to get it all out of my system. The anger, the resentment, the bitterness, the 'Poor-Me's' all had to be given time to drain away. I felt so let down by him. I felt so sorry for myself and kept asking myself what I had done to deserve this. I found it was such hard work trying to fathom him out. Now I don't waste my time and energy trying to get inside his head. I've learned that in this group. I've learned how to cope in here.

I've learned that any work I put into trying to fathom anyone out should be focused on myself and my own survival. I've finally started to take my hands off my alcoholic and be my own best friend and not to rely on him for my own happiness."

Clarissa stops again and struggles to compose herself and hold back the tears.

"Now I know I always have a bolt-hole to go to. I am not carrying this enormous weight on my own anymore. I have a steel ladder, not a wooden one, to help me climb out of the black pit I was in. I became so sick because I was too focused on him and had let every other part of my life go.

My self-esteem, had all drained away and I was totally exhausted. Although I still loved my husband and wanted to fix him I did feel like a victim just waiting for the next bomb to go off. I always felt very lonely because I could not go to him for help or support and I was angry about that. If I told him any of my secrets he would just blurt them all out in public when he was over the knot.

One day it just all became too much and I told him to get out and stay out. I thought by kicking him out it would bring him to his senses. I thought once he realised he stood to lose his wife and kids he would put the drink down."

She laughs.

"Well I can laugh about that now because it seems so ridiculous but at the time that was the extent of my master plan! What really happened was he was as 'happy as Larry' because he finally had no one on his back all the time telling him not to drink. He was free to just get on and drink 24/7 and at first he just got even worse!

My anxiety levels went through the roof and I had three young children who I had sole responsibility for and I was like a raging banshee. I dread to think what damage I caused to my kids emotional well-being during that time.

I knew I needed help but I didn't know where to get it. I bought books written by so called experts and watched any snippets there were on telly but I felt that at the end of the day I was really just left to try and sort it all out by myself. My doctor told me to just leave him for good because there wasn't any medication that could cure him, he would always be a drunk. But my doctor didn't tell me there was something out there for me. He didn't tell me about this support group.

It wasn't until I confided in someone at my Sociology class that I was told about AL and even then it took me months to build up the courage to come along to a meeting. Several times I drove past but just couldn't bring myself to come in. One night after yet another bust-up with my husband I just stormed through those doors using my anger to fuel me. Thank goodness I did. I know he has picked up again but . . ."

Clarissa's voice starts to falter but she continues . . .

"Coming to AL has improved my life no end. I have had to learn to change my ways of thinking. I am a lot stronger now. I do know this programme is not bullet proof and I know it doesn't stop bad things happening but it's the best thing I've found for helping me to cope with life.

I'm grateful because 'Mrs Next-Door' hasn't got this programme and I wouldn't like to go back to being in that position again. It works for me and that's why I keep coming back.

Thank you."

GROUP TOGETHER

"Thanks Clarissa"

JEFF

"I'll come in Mack."

Jeff is a man of around 55, he has always prided himself on his ability to solve problems. He feels he shouldn't have to come to a place like AL but accepts it as his last port of call in learning how to cope with his alcoholic son.

"Well it's my son who is the alcoholic in my life and I came to AL because for the first time in my life I found I didn't have all the answers. I've never liked to look at anything bad. I've only ever wanted to look at the good and the positive. I've just always moved forwards and never looked back on the results of any of my actions. When this problem came into my life I had no answers as to how to deal with it. I still don't have many answers and that's why I keep coming back I'm still looking for the answers."

Jeff clenches his jaw and shrugs his shoulders to indicate that he has finished his share.

GROUP TOGETHER

"Thanks Jeff."

Mack looks up at the clock on the wall and registers surprise.

<u>MACK</u>

"Well we have 2 minutes left of the meeting if anyone would like to come in with a short share."

<u>JOSH</u>

"I would just like to say thank you to everyone for what I have heard tonight. I shall go home and think over everything I've heard because it's a bit hard to think about it all now. But thank you all anyway."

<u>GROUP TOGETHER</u>

"Thanks Josh."

<u>MACK</u>

"Oh, one thing I forgot to mention to our newcomers is that we suggest you come back for at least 6 meetings before you decide whether it's for you or not. The reason we say that is because we have different members and different topics here at different times and it could be that you don't find anyone you feel you can identify with at your first few meetings. However, if after 6 meetings you find no identification then the group is probably either not for you or not for you at this time.

Before we close our meeting tonight I will just remind everybody that the topic for the next meeting is:

Detachment from the problem

Do we have a volunteer to be the main sharer for next time?"

There is a long pause

<u>VICKY</u>

"I will be the main sharer Mack."

MACK

"Thank You Vicky.

So it just remains for me to say for the benefit of our newcomers that there are no dues for membership but we do ask you to make a contribution of whatever you can afford to cover our costs for tea and coffee and rent. If you cannot afford anything then that is OK too.

OK, I'm afraid our time is up and we close on time, so Stavros, can I ask you to read the suggested closing to close our meeting?"

STAVROS

"In closing, I would like to say that the opinions expressed here were strictly those of the person who gave them. Take what you liked and leave the rest. A few words to those of you who haven't been with us long: whatever your problems, there are those amongst us who have had them too. If you try to keep an open mind, you will find help. You will come to realise that there is no situation too difficult to be bettered and no unhappiness too great to be lessened.

Will all those who care to join me in closing our meeting?"

Everyone joins hands in a circle.

GROUP TOGETHER

"Grant me the Serenity to accept the things I cannot change.

The courage to change the things I can and

The wisdom to know the difference.

Same time, Same Place, Keep coming back, it works if you work it."

Meeting 2

Tonight's Topic—Detachment from the problem

ELSA says,

"Ok, shall we begin the meeting?

One of the disciplines in AL is that we start on time and we finish on time, regardless.

So, I will read the suggested opening:

We would like to welcome you to this AL meeting.

The AL meeting is a group of relatives and friends of problem drinkers who share their experience, strength and hope in order to solve their common problems. We believe alcoholism is a family illness and that changed attitudes can aid recovery.

For the benefit of Pippa, who is here tonight, I would like to go round the room and introduce ourselves, using first names only and if anyone chooses to, they can say who the problem drinker is in their lives."

Meet the Group

ELSA

"OK, I will start with myself—Hello, I'm Elsa and I am chairing the meeting tonight. I am an adult child of an alcoholic (ACOA). The alcoholic in my life is my father."

CLARISSA

"Hello, my name is Clarissa the alcoholic in my life is my husband. He's very up and down at the moment so I am trying my hardest to emotionally detach from his behaviour. I am here tonight for me."

VICKY

"Hello, my name is Vicky and the problem drinker in my life is my daughter."

FADIA

"Hello my name is Fadia and I have been affected by my grandfather's drinking. When I was young I was sent to live with my grandparents and found myself caught up in the chaos caused by his drinking."

KALEB

"Hello, I'm Kaleb and my wife is the drinker in my life. I haven't been coming here long but my life has definitely got easier over the past few months."

EDDIE

"Well I'm Eddie and as most of you know I'm a 'double-winner'. For Pippa's benefit that simply means I'm a member of two support groups. I'm a recovering alcoholic myself but I'm also married to a recovering alcoholic so I qualify for membership of AL too."

JOSH

"Hello, my name's Josh and this is only my second meeting."

JEFF

"My name is Jeff and the person with the drink problem in my life is my son."

STAVROS

"Hello, I'm Stavros and the person with the drink problem was my wife."

INGRID

"I'm Ingrid and I was at the last meeting. I have already begun to feel better since coming here."

ALICE

"Hello, I'm Alice and I'm married to Jeff. We come along to the meeting together because it's our son who has a drink problem."

PIPPA

"Hello, I'm Pippa and I am back tonight because I feel I need help to get through a crisis I have going on in my life right now. I came to AL about two years ago but left after 3 meetings. I thought I didn't need to come here because my partner got himself into AA and I thought everything would be fine after that but it wasn't and I left him last weekend and am temporarily sleeping on a friend's sofa until I find a flat."

ELSA

"Welcome back Pippa."

Elsa is chairing the meeting tonight and is a woman in her mid-50's. She is the adult child of an alcoholic. The alcoholic in her life is her father. Elsa is a long time member.

"It may all still seem very strange at first and you will probably go away not understanding much about what you hear tonight but if you feel something that brings you back then that is enough to be going on with. Just keep coming back and it will eventually all start to become much clearer about what support is on offer here.

Can I remind everyone that this is an anonymous group and we use first names only. Anonymity is one of the key principles we adhere to in the group. You do not need to tell us who you are, where you live, where you work, what you do—absolutely nothing about your personal details at all if you don't want to.

There are 12 of us here tonight but the numbers vary each week and sometimes there are more of us and sometimes less.

You don't have to come every week but we do suggest you attend as regularly as you possibly can if you want to benefit from what's on offer. Our only reason for being here is to share our experience, strength and hope to help ourselves and each other to gain some peace of mind because our lives have been impacted on by somebody with an alcohol problem. Anything else about your life is no concern of ours unless you choose to share it with us.

So, as I've said my name is Elsa and although I am chairing the meeting tonight, next time someone else will be chairing because we practice the principle of rotation of leadership in the group.

Also, although we meet up in a church hall this programme is not religious and has no connection to any church. The only reason we meet here is because of low costs.

So on with the meeting. Every week we have a different theme and tonight's theme is:

Detachment—how do I do it?

Clarissa can you start us off with the 12 steps please?"

CLARISSA

"**Step 1**: We admitted we were powerless over the problem drinker and that our lives had become unmanageable."

VICKY

"**Step 2**: We came to believe that a power greater than ourselves could restore us to serenity."

FADIA

"**Step 3**: We made a decision to turn our will and our lives over to the care of our higher power (HP)."

KALEB

"**Step 4:** We made a searching and fearless moral inventory of ourselves."

EDDIE

"**Step 5:** We admitted to our HP, to ourselves and to another human being the exact nature of our wrongs."

JOSH

"**Step 6:** We were entirely ready to have our HP remove all these defects of character."

JEFF

"**Step 7:** We humbly asked our HP to remove our shortcomings."

STAVROS

"**Step 8:** We made a list of all persons we had harmed and became willing to make amends to them all."

INGRID

"**Step 9:** We made direct amends to such people wherever possible, except when to do so would injure them or others."

ALICE

"**Step 10:** We continued to take personal inventory and when we were wrong promptly admitted it."

PIPPA

"**Step 11:** We sought through reflection and meditation to improve our conscious contact with our HP, seeking only knowledge of our HP's will for us and the power to carry that out."

ELSA

"**Step 12:** Having had an emotional and spiritual awakening as the result of these Steps, we tried to carry this message to others, and to practice these principles in all our affairs.

Vicky has agreed to be our main sharer tonight and can I just remind you that there is no obligation for anyone to share. You can remain silent and just listen if you want but those who do decide to share are allowed to do so without interruption from anyone else.

So over to you Vicky, on the theme of:

Detachment—how do I do it?"

Vicky is a relatively recent member of AL but she has spent a couple of years chaperoning her daughter to AA meetings.

VICKY

"Thank you Elsa and thank you all for being here tonight. I think out of all the things which the programme helps me to deal with I find this one the hardest thing to do. To practice detachment is hard and for me, I think because it is my child it is doubly hard. I have to say this is also quite a painful subject because it caused a lot of trouble and fighting in our house because of my absolute refusal and inability to detach from the problem.

My husband had always been there for me as my best friend, my right arm really and then this problem of alcoholism came into our lives and it was awful. I felt I could no longer depend on him because I had my ideas and he had his about what was the best way to deal with the turmoil we found ourselves in. I was stuck in the now and wanted to do things just to put everything right with her, I thought I would get our daughter put right and everything would get back to normal again. I took her to AA meetings for two years and sat with her thinking I was 'Mrs Super-Mum' but my husband could see further ahead than me, he could see things were not going to return to the way they were before all of this started.

I think another reason why I had great difficulty detaching was because at the back of my mind I felt as if we were abandoning our daughter and my husband didn't see it that way at all, so there were huge rows at home it was a very stressful time and it took a long while but eventually, it was the strength of this programme that helped me to see things more clearly.

The next problem was how much detachment? What did detachment mean for us because detachment means different things to different people. To my husband it meant he didn't want anything to do with our daughter at all while she was still drinking. He didn't want to see her, he didn't want to hear about her. That was it. End of story. She really didn't exist for him. Whereas, I couldn't do that, I still had to know what she was up to and any news I got of her felt like a life-line to me.

Yes, to emotionally step-back was the right thing to do but I feel as if I would have liked a bit more contact but the matter was taken out of our hands by our daughter. She just took off one day and we didn't see her for almost a year. She decided she wanted no contact with us and none of her friends would tell us where she was living. Thankfully we are in contact today and our relationship is OK'ish so we must have handled it alright. I find I need the programme to help me to keep getting the balance right.

When I first heard the word detachment I thought it meant putting a wall up and having no contact at all and just trying to put her completely out of my mind. I think learning to detach emotionally but not physically is very possible for me once I have learned how to manage not getting too pulled into her problem, which I am having to practice again this week because she has started drinking again.

I think I'm getting better at detaching and how I manage it is by still having some contact but emotionally detaching and not getting so involved in her problem. Detachment to me doesn't mean I don't care for her but that I care equally for myself and I have a responsibility to take care of myself too. What I had called love was really just me trying to fix her to sooth my own levels of anxiety instead of seeing her as a separate person who can make her own choices even if those choices are not the same as mine.

So for me detachment has been about learning to have boundaries, making rules really and trying to stick to them but it is so difficult to do, in fact, it can sometimes be nigh on impossible. It reminds me of one day when our daughter was living with us and she took herself off to the town and got mortal drunk and we got a phone call from the police and they were really indignant because we wouldn't go down and get her and bring her home. My husband was adamant he wasn't going to get her because he said he had had enough of it over the last 5 years, so this policeman said "what do you expect we are going to do with her?" and my husband told him to do whatever he would do with any drunk that he found lying in the town square. So our daughter ended up sleeping it off in the cells. So that is one example of us being tested to the absolute limit and still trying to cling on to the few boundaries we had put in place to try to protect our own sanity.

I have learned in the group not to expect detachment to be a quick process and not to expect to be able to do it perfectly the first time around. For me it's been about taking tiny steps back, one by one, until enough distance is created to allow me to focus sufficiently on my own life too. I have found the slogan *'Easy Does It'* to be very helpful in reminding myself that detachment for me is best if it is a slow and gradual process. It was suggested in here that the alcoholic would resist me detaching every inch of the way and I have found that to be true—she doesn't want me to *'Let Go'* of her really. I try to distance myself from her words, her feelings and her actions when she has been drinking. One minute she wants me doing things for her that she should really be doing for herself and the next minute she accuses me of being controlling and domineering, so I found from experience that I was an easy target for emotional manipulation, so detachment is proving to be a mental and emotional safety-net for me.

I have set goal-posts and I have tried to keep to them but our daughter has chipped away at them time and time again and each time she tries to pull me a bit further into her own alcoholic problems but I soon realise it now and I make more efforts to slowly keep stepping back and allowing her to pick up the consequences of her actions for herself.

Looking back I would say my recovery started the moment I started to practice detaching from her and I've consciously changed my attitude towards giving her advice. I now think to myself, how do I really know what is best for her? How can I be sure I have the right answers for her life? How do I know what her path is? Once I started to ask myself these questions I realised that the truth is I don't know all the answers for her so I should leave her to make her own decisions.

I now see detachment as a way of showing my daughter respect and it also lets her see that I have had a change of attitude and maybe, just maybe she might feel the need to make some changes of her own. I felt as if we were in a kind of nightmare dance that wasn't doing either of us any good. I was waiting for her to change so the dance would end but she didn't change and things just went round and round in circles and progressively got worse taking both of us down with it. I suppose I used the slogan *'Change—Let it begin with me'* and I have changed, so the dance has changed too and although I still feel as if I have a long way to go I do feel it is no longer the insane, emotional rollercoaster that it once was.

My life is more peaceful today. I do have joy back in my life. Yes, there are still grey days but I feel the programme is giving me a training in how to manage my own emotions so that I don't allow myself to be so easily manipulated by the alcoholic. I do have conscious choices today. I can distance myself from her unacceptable behaviour and not allow her to provoke frustration, anger, resentment and even depression in me. I can grant her less accessibility to my emotions and make a conscious choice to give less by reminding myself of the negative consequences it causes in my own life if I give too much.

I think to a large extent it also had something to do with pride as well, I simply refused to admit defeat. I was going to fix-her if it was the last thing I did and it very nearly was the last thing I ever did. Unfortunately, I became a victim of my own obsession to fix her and was almost driven insane because of it.

I have had to learn about detachment because I had no idea how to detach before I came to AL. With the benefit of hindsight I can now see that I'd never been able to step-back and let our daughter make her own choices. I wanted her to do what I wanted. It's only by learning from everyone else's experience, strength and hope that I have gained the ability to end my struggling and accept that it's her problem not mine and that she has to deal with it in her own way.

I have found saying No to people very difficult because saying No to some people is almost like a slap in the face. So I think how I say No makes a big difference too. If I say it in a harsh tone or in a hostile reaction mode it just fans the flames and causes me more trouble but if I say 'No—I wouldn't feel comfortable with that' it seems to be more acceptable to not only my daughter but to most people. So for me it's all about detachment with love and compassion not detachment with anger, hostility and resentment.

So I will just end by saying detachment works for me so I will continue to practice it—and thank you everybody for being here tonight and for all the help you have given me to get through this."

GROUP TOGETHER

"Thanks Vicky."

FADIA

"Can I come in Elsa?"

Fadia has been in the group for some time and can speak in a way which reveals her years of experience of sharing her feelings.

"Thank you Vicky for your share I got a lot out of that. I would like to mention the feelings of guilt I got when I first started detaching from my grandparents. I felt as if I should be so grateful to them for bringing me up when my own parents had sent me from Morocco to live with them. I felt as if I should just allow their needs to take priority over mine and I realise now I just settled for being their carer really. It was a role-reversal of sorts because I never felt I could be a child and just be carefree and spontaneous, I always felt I owed them.

My grandfather was a binge drinker and would be very argumentative in drink and although my grandmother got the brunt of it, just being there and watching it all going on and feeling responsible in some way was a very heavy burden for me as a child to take on. Once I got into AL I began to see how I had just been enabling the situation to continue by catering to everyone else's needs in an attempt to keep the peace. I had long since taken the focus off my own life and my own ambitions.

When I moved out and got a bed-sit of my own the guilt was overwhelming. I kept going back two or three times a week just to sit and listen to my grandmother's endless rants about the disappointments she had had in her life, who she could have married and didn't, what she could have been and wasn't—she was very negative and stuck in a rut really. But it did make me feel less guilty and that was the price I was prepared to pay because I think a more rapid or hostile detachment for me would have been just too painful

36

to do. So very, very slowly was how I did my detachment so I could get used to my new freedom and slowly build an independent life for myself away from the alcoholic environment I had been brought up in. An environment I had loved in my own naive way for so long because I had known no different.

I had never learned how to stand back before coming into AL. My instinct had always told me to move forward, closer to the problem and try to solve it and that attitude is fine if it is a problem I can solve, but if it's a problem I can't solve then what? The truth is my own attitude had caused me a lot of unnecessary suffering because I couldn't discern which problems I could solve from those I couldn't so I was caught up in a vicious circle for a long time. It was only when I came here and saw how others had managed to get off the 'roundabout' and make their lives better, that I felt I had some hope of being able to do the same. One of the tools I used was the Serenity Prayer—'Grant me the serenity to accept the things I cannot change, the courage to change the things I can and the wisdom to know the difference' and I thank you all for pointing me in the right direction of detaching with love, it has definitely changed my life for the better."

GROUP TOGETHER

"Thanks Fadia."

EDDIE

"I will just come in if you like Elsa."

Eddie is an alcoholic and has been a member of AA for 20 years. He has been sober for 18 years. He is a semi-retired university lecturer. He joined AL 18 months ago.

"Well detachment for me just means Step 1 really, which is my acceptance of my powerlessness over another person's drinking. It now seems like an obvious thing but it took me quite a long time for it to finally dawn on me. It sounds like a simple thing, standing—back, it should be very easy to do but it's not because for a long time I have had this way of life where I thought I knew best. I thought I could keep everything right and I could tell my wife what to do but she is not a kid and I have learned in AL that she has every right to do whatever she wants but if she comes to me and asks me what I think then I am quite happy to tell her but it's not my job to just tell her and try to keep her right without her asking for my input. It's about accepting that I am powerless over anybody else's life.

If someone wants to make a mess of their lives and 'active' alcoholics inevitably do make a mess of things that's their prerogative really and I can understand, Vicky, how that tears a parent apart because we are naturally programmed to want to 'micro manage' our children but the reality of the situation is we truly have no more control over our children than we have over any other human being. I am powerless over anybody else's life, including my wife's. It's just taken me a very long time to be able to get my head around that and I have had to learn to stop doing the things I always used to do because that is just what I have always done.

So practicing detachment has led to a new way of life for me and I know for a fact if I had continued with my old behaviour I would have just got the same results of the old unmanageability and chaos that brought me to AL in the first place. For me I try to keep everything as simple as I can using the slogan *'Keep it Simple'* because I find it stops me tipping over into obsessive thinking again.

I am not saying it is easy because I know it isn't easy, it remains something I have to be constantly aware of and the solution for me is not just cold detachment because I do love my wife dearly but she is entitled to make a mess of her life or even a triumph of it. It's up to her, it's not my job to live her life for her. Also for me when I am powerless it's about having trust and faith that she has a HP of her own who she can call upon to guide her. She also has AA and the people there who have walked this path before her, who can share their experience, strength and hope.

When I first started practising detachment, my wife accused me of being cold and disinterested but I wasn't unconcerned I was just emotionally stepping back a bit. In AA it is suggested that if you find yourself in a situation you cannot handle very well get out of the situation. If I stay I'm an 'aunt sally' and if I leave the room she says to me "Oh yes, that's you running away again". It is difficult because I am partly dependent on her because she is my wife and that is what marriage is about.

When I see her going to make mistakes that I had already made, been there, got the T-shirt, sort of thing, I would say don't do that because I didn't want her to make the same mistakes I had made and get into all the difficulties that I did, not because I wanted to dominate her but because I wanted to help her. And she misinterprets that as dominating. It's not about dominance, I wanted her to do things differently because it would help her—but I have got a lot of anger and resentment back for that. It's very complicated from where I am sitting at the moment. I do feel it's about getting the balance right and I also feel as if I am very much still working on this.

I'll just leave it at that thanks Elsa."

GROUP TOGETHER

"Thanks Eddie."

INGRID

"Can I come in Elsa?"

Last week was Ingrid's first AL meeting. It's her husband who is alcohol dependant.

"I've tried detaching several times by leaving my husband and going back to my mother's but I have always ended up going back because he needs me to look after him. When we were living in separate houses I found I may as well have been living with him because although we were physically apart he was still living in my head all the time anyway.

He just seems to know how to press all of my emotional buttons and I find myself on an enormous guilt trip if I don't drop everything and go running to help him. He has me believing he drinks because I nag him so much. I feel he messes about with my head and always manages to manoeuvre me into a position of putting his needs to the top of the pile and my needs fly out of the window. I then get so annoyed and angry with myself for not standing my ground but I can't seem to find my own way out of this toxic dance we seem to have going on.

This is only my second meeting but already I have felt a shift in my attitude towards him so that's why I'm back tonight. I feel I need all the support I can get because my doctor has told me I have to start looking after myself and reduce my stress levels. So coming here—is me standing up for myself for once and that makes me feel better already."

GROUP TOGETHER

"Thanks Ingrid."

PIPPA

"Can I just say a few words Elsa?

I don't think I will be able to get much out tonight but here goes . . ."

Pippa attended a few AL meetings last year but decided it wasn't for her. She's come back today because she has recently left her alcoholic boyfriend and is sleeping on a friend's sofa. She feels at this time she needs the support of the group.

"I left my partner last weekend and I'm staying with a friend.

I've decided I've just had enough."

Pippa pauses trying to compose herself before continuing.

"I think listening to everybody tonight—it seems to be really hard to keep boundaries and keep my emotions pinned down when I am living 24hrs a day with someone who is drinking. Now I'm thinking about what I want because I've never thought about what I wanted. All my energy has been taken up just trying to keep things OK in the house. I've spent most of my time searching for bottles and pouring booze down the sink or watering it down so he won't drink so much but he just finds another hiding place. It's like cat and mouse really.

Money has got so tight—I'm having to borrow from my parents just to keep afloat. Really I suppose I've just become obsessed with trying to change him into the man I want him to be. He says the most hurtful things to me and I try to just ignore his words but I end up wondering if there is any truth in them. I have clung on to one slogan I got from my first visit a couple of years ago and that is *'I didn't cause it, I can't control it and I can't cure it'.* That slogan has come back to me time and time again when I have been in the depths of despair. It has given me great comfort to be told in here that I didn't cause his drinking because he always tells me all of this is my fault.

It seems like no matter what I did, whatever happened, even if I knew deep down I was right it would be turned around so I wasn't right, so I never felt secure in thinking well yes I can go down that road because I know that will work out. There was always something at the back of my mind saying, 'Hey what are you doing? That might be wrong'. So I never had the confidence to see things through. I know I am changing because at one time I would never say No. I'm saying No now by moving out but it is leaving me with awful feelings of grief and guilt, even failure.

I went to see a flat today and I thought oh, am I going to be living here? It's really getting to me. Trying to change things is tough and I find I have to keep writing notes to myself to motivate me to do

41

anything. I'm really grateful to have somewhere to come to tonight and get all of this off my chest. I do feel as if you all know where I am coming from and I don't have to justify myself. I can't tell you what a relief that is.

Thank you."

GROUP TOGETHER

"Thanks Pippa."

ALICE

"I'll come in Elsa."

Alice is married to Jeff. They come along to the meetings together because their son is an alcoholic who is drunk most days.

"Well, really I don't do detachment very well but I've made huge improvements compared with what I was when I first came here. When I first came to AL I didn't have a life anymore but with everyone's help and support I feel I've now started to live my own life again. I do try to put goal-posts in place and I made a rule that our son had to be sober when he comes to our house. If he's the worse for drink I put him in a taxi and send him home."

Alice pauses for a moment as if she has lost the thread of her thinking, then turning to Pippa she continues.

"And can I just say to Pippa, don't be too hard on yourself because it is especially tough living under the same roof with an alcoholic. Our son nearly drove us both round the bend when we had him living with us and although it can still be very stressful seeing him three times a week it is nothing like as bad as it was when we had him living in our house with us."

Alice picks up the original thread of her share again.

"I suppose our first stepping-stone towards detachment was when we gave him an ultimatum, either he stopped drinking or he had to move out and find his own place, to our absolute amazement he chose to move out and it wasn't until he'd left that we really began to see just how much we had missed out on having a peaceful home to live in.

Now where the main trouble lies for me is when he's drunk and the phone calls start. He rings, asking me to go for alcohol and when I refuse he starts by saying please, then he progresses on to pleading and then he ends up by begging down the phone. I say no for a while and then I say no again, but eventually I get absolutely worn-down and plagued with his non-stop phoning that I end up taking the phone out of the socket and then I start worrying because he has got himself into some very bad states in the past and anyone else who did that would be in hospital. Then he promises he will give it up if I go round but nine times out of ten before we even get from his house to mine he is demanding a detour to the off-licence to get more alcohol and then he will say it's just for tonight and I will stop in the morning and yep I've fallen for it again. Then I get really annoyed with myself for caving in. But then I rationalise it and tell myself someone has to go for his booze because he is so ill he can't walk to the shops himself. In fact, he can't walk anywhere, he can't walk down the stairs so he does depend on me to go for it. It happens every time and every time I tell myself I have got to have a rule where I just refuse to go and stick to my boundaries but I haven't got there yet.

I keep telling myself I have just got to be strong enough to keep saying no but I find that very hard because he is breaking my heart and he's crying and moaning and saying he's going to die and all of that crap comes out and then if I say no he starts threatening to bang on his neighbours door and ask them to get him some booze. So I go round just to keep the peace so that's the bit I have got to get over.

With regards to detaching emotionally I try to but I am sad. Whereas before I would have been inconsolable, absolutely devastated even, but I am not now, I am sad. I do still have to learn to keep to that boundary of not letting him wrong foot me with sentimentality and remind myself that it is his responsibility, he is the one pouring it down his throat not me and if I'm buying it for him, I am really just helping him to kill himself.

Sorry if that sounded like a bit of a rant but he still really gets to me so I'll just stop for now.

Thank you."

GROUP TOGETHER

"Thanks Alice."

KALEB

"I'll share Elsa."

Kaleb's wife is the problem drinker in his life. Kaleb has only been coming to AL for the past few months and although he is in the early stages of recovery, he is already starting to feel the benefits of the group.

"Detachment is not something I have really practised a lot until this past year I think and I have found it to be a very good tool. I think for me detachment is all about standing back from my wife's behaviour and thinking about things and not just launching in with my quick-fix solutions, which may not be the best way to go anyway. Maybe it is the right route for her, maybe she should be doing what she is doing, I don't know. Maybe there is a different way, a better way she could go than just doing what I think she should do. It's about not allowing myself to get drawn into all the upset and emotional dramas.

I try to be as calm as possible and it feels much better doing that than how I used to react with anger in the past. Now I detach from a lot of the emotional stuff that is thrown at me, which becomes even more difficult to deal with if I just react. It's about being able to detach from my own emotions enough to be able to look at them and allow myself to make a conscious choice as to how I am going to respond to any given crisis without denying to myself that the alcohol problem exists.

This thing with boundaries, I find it very difficult to put boundaries in place in my house. It is virtually impossible, if you are living with somebody who is also the co-owner of the house, to say no they cannot come into their own house when they have been drinking too much but maybe I should have some courage to change rather than just leaving things unsaid, I am still working on that one. I do think boundaries can be a good source of communication because it is a way of saying look I am serious now, I don't want this unacceptable behaviour to continue, but so far I haven't been able to do it. I think I am still hankering after a peaceful life too much. I think I sometimes still detach with a sort of indifference, rather than with love or compassion, especially when it all just becomes too much for me to process and deal with at the time, so I just push the problem right out of my mind for a while to save my own sanity.

And that's all I want to say for now."

GROUP TOGETHER

"Thanks Kaleb."

CLARISSA

"I'll come in Elsa."

Clarissa is a women in her mid 30's with 3 young children and an alcoholic husband who is in AA.

"Can I just start by saying welcome to Pippa, it's lovely to see you back because I know how difficult it is to walk through those doors and ask for help.

As you all know the alcoholic in my life is my husband and he is back off the booze at the moment and working his own programme in AA tonight so I am grateful for that.

I can understand what's been said about detaching emotionally because if I had not done that with my husband I would definitely have gone over the edge. I really would have because the emotional battering I got off him with his continual confrontations was an on-going source of pain for me, he'd act and I'd react and my reaction becomes a justification for him drinking again. So I did manage to cut off from him but it was sad really looking back on it now because I realised he was not going to change and I detached with resentment just to stop me getting all of this aggravation from him.

I did feel rejected when he would not accept my help. I detached by building this wall around myself to protect me because there was only so much I could take and then this self-protective instinct kicked-in. He has since told me it was the best thing I had ever done for him because he knew he had no one else to depend on and nowhere else to go so he had to make some major changes in his life. I found it much easier to emotionally detach from him once things had gone past a critical point, I just knew my own wellbeing was in danger.

I suppose the reason it took me so long was because I didn't really want to detach. It can feel very isolating for me too and I don't want to be that isolated from another human being, but I still have to protect myself emotionally because if I go over the edge how is that going to help the situation at all.

I don't know whether any of that made sense but I'll just stop there for now."

GROUP TOGETHER

"Thanks Clarissa."

Elsa looks up at the clock on the wall and sees the time is almost up.

ELSA

"Well we have 5 minutes left of the meeting if anyone would like to come in with a short share?"

JOSH

"I will just say a few words Elsa."

Josh is a medical student. The drinker in his life was his twin sister. She died last year. This is Josh's second meeting.

"Detachment is a strange subject for me because my sister died so I have been forced into being permanently separated from her but I did take on board what has been said about her still living in my head and that is absolutely true because there isn't a day goes by when I don't think of her. I think I have joined the group because I'm looking for answers. I want to know more about this illness and why my sister had it and was there anything I could have done differently which would have helped. I suppose I feel guilty that I wasn't able to save her."

Josh shows signs of becoming overcome with emotion and stops speaking for a while.

"That's all I feel I can say at the moment."

GROUP TOGETHER

"Thanks Josh."

ELSA

"Can I also just say to Pippa we suggest you come back for at least 6 meetings before you decide whether it's for you or not. The reason we say that is because we have different members and different topics here at different times and it could be that you don't find anyone you feel you can identify with at your first few meetings.

However, if after 6 meetings you find no identification then the group is probably either not for you or not for you at this time.

Before we close our meeting tonight I will just remind everybody that the theme for next time is:

Self-Esteem

Do we have a volunteer to be the main sharer for next time?"

There is a short pause.

INGRID

"I will be the main sharer Elsa."

ELSA

"Thank You Ingrid.

So it just remains for me to say for the benefit of our newcomers that there are no dues for membership but we do ask you to make a contribution of whatever you can afford to cover our costs for tea and coffee and rent. If you cannot afford anything then that is OK too.

OK, I'm afraid our time is up and we close on time, so Kaleb, can I ask you to read the suggested closing to close our meeting please?"

KALEB

"In closing, I would like to say that the opinions expressed here were strictly those of the person who gave them. Take what you liked and leave the rest. A few words to those of you who haven't been with us long: whatever your problems, there are those amongst us who have had them too. If you try to keep an open mind, you will find help. You will come to realise that there is no situation too difficult to be bettered and no unhappiness too great to be lessened.

Will all those who care to join me in closing our meeting?"

Everyone joins hands in a circle.

GROUP TOGETHER

"Grant me the Serenity to accept the things I cannot change.

The courage to change the things I can and

The wisdom to know the difference.

Same time, Same Place, Keep coming back, it works if you work it."

Meeting 3

Tonight's Topic—Self-esteem

FADIA says,

"Ok, shall we make a start everybody?

One of the disciplines in AL is that we start on time and we finish on time, regardless.

So, I will read the suggested opening:

We would like to welcome you to this AL meeting.

The AL meeting is a group of relatives and friends of problem drinkers who share their experience, strength and hope in order to solve their common problems. We believe alcoholism is a family illness and that changed attitudes can aid recovery.

Although we have no newcomers here tonight I would still like us to go round the room and introduce ourselves, using first names only because it's still early days for Josh, Ingrid and Pippa and it takes us all a little time to remember everybody's name."

Meet the Group

FADIA

"OK, I will start with me—I'm Fadia and I am chairing the meeting tonight. I am an adult child of an alcoholic (ACOA). The alcoholic in my life was my grandfather who I lived with when I was a child."

CLARISSA

"Hello, I'm Clarissa and the alcoholic in my life is my husband but I am here tonight for me."

VICKY

"Hello, I'm Vicky and the problem drinker in my life is my daughter."

EDDIE

"I'm Eddie and as you all know I'm a 'double-winner'—a member of two support groups. I'm a recovering alcoholic but I'm also married to a recovering alcoholic so I qualify for membership of AL too as I have a family member who is an alcoholic."

JOSH

"Hello, my name's Josh and this is my third meeting."

JEFF

"My name is Jeff and the person with the drink problem in our life is our son. My wife Alice usually comes along to this meeting with me but tonight she's gone to a school reunion dinner so she isn't here tonight. Our son is still drinking."

STAVROS

"Hello, I'm Stavros and the person with the alcohol problem was my wife."

INGRID

"I'm Ingrid and this is my third meeting and I have offered to be the main sharer for tonight. I have already started to feel much better since coming here."

PIPPA

"Hello, I'm Pippa and I am back tonight because I feel I need help to get through my current crisis with my partner. I am still sleeping on a friend's sofa until I find a flat I haven't buckled under yet even though he's been ringing me all week blaming me for his drinking problems."

MACK

"Hi, I'm Mack and it's my son who is addicted to alcohol."

ELSA

"Hello I'm Elsa and I am a long time member of the group and it is my father who is the alcoholic in my life."

FADIA

"A special word for Pippa, Josh and Ingrid."

Fadia is chairing the meeting tonight. She is a woman in her 20's and is the adult child of an alcoholic. The alcoholic in her life was her grandfather. Fadia is a long-time member of AL.

"Welcome back—it may all still seem strange and you will probably go away not understanding much about what you hear tonight but if you feel something that brings you back then that is enough to be going on with. Just keep coming back and it will eventually start to become much clearer about what support you can gain from the group.

Can I remind everyone that this is an anonymous group and we use first names only. Anonymity is one of the key principles we adhere to in the group.

You do not need to tell us who you are, where you live, where you work, what you do—absolutely nothing about your personal details at all if you don't want to.

There are 11 of us here tonight but the numbers vary each week and sometimes there are more of us and sometimes less.

You don't have to come every week but we do suggest you attend as regularly as you can if you want to benefit from what's on offer here. Our only purpose is to share our experience, strength and hope to help ourselves and each other to gain some peace of mind because our lives have been affected by an alcoholic dependant person. Anything else about your life is no concern of ours unless you choose to share it with us.

So, as I've said my name is Fadia and although I am chairing the meeting tonight, next time someone else will be chairing because we practice the principle of rotation of leadership in the group.

Also, although we meet up in a church hall this programme is not religious and has no connection to any church. The only reason we meet here is because of low costs.

So on with the meeting. Every week we have a different theme and tonight's theme is:

Self-Esteem

Jeff can you start us off with the 12 steps please?"

JEFF

Step 1: We admitted we were powerless over the problem drinker and that our lives had become unmanageable."

STAVROS

Step 2: We came to believe that a power greater than ourselves could restore us to serenity."

INGRID

Step 3: We made a decision to turn our will and our lives over to the care of our higher power (HP)."

PIPPA

Step 4: We made a searching and fearless moral inventory of ourselves."

MACK

Step 5: We admitted to our HP, to ourselves and to another human being the exact nature of our wrongs."

ELSA

Step 6: We were entirely ready to have our HP remove all these defects of character."

FADIA

Step 7: We humbly asked our HP to remove our shortcomings."

CLARISSA

Step 8: We made a list of all persons we had harmed and became willing to make amends to them all."

VICKY

Step 9: We made direct amends to such people wherever possible, except when to do so would injure them or others."

EDDIE

Step 10: We continued to take personal inventory and when we were wrong promptly admitted it."

JOSH

"Step 11: We sought through reflection and meditation to improve our conscious contact with our HP, seeking only knowledge of our HP's will for us and the power to carry that out."

JEFF

"Step 12: Having had an emotional and spiritual awakening as the result of these Steps, we tried to carry this message to others, and to practice these principles in all our affairs."

FADIA

"Ingrid has agreed to be our main sharer for tonight and can I just remind you that there is no obligation for anyone to share. You can remain silent and just listen if you prefer but those who do decide to share are allowed to do so without interruption from others.

So over to you Ingrid, on the theme of:

Self-esteem"

Ingrid's husband is alcohol dependant. She is concerned how having alcoholism in the family has affected the lives of her and her children. As Ingrid is still only a very recent member of AL, she is still very emotional when she shares her experiences with the group.

INGRID

"This is a hard one for me because I was this outgoing, confident person—bubbly, really good at my job but then alcoholism came into my life. I lost all my self-esteem due to the stress, the worry, the anger and all of those negative habits I developed from being in this situation. At one time I could go into any social situation and mix with any company but now I find it difficult. Sometimes I find it difficult to join in and at other times I can be a bit over the top by just pretending to be having a good time.

I think I also lost my self-esteem along the way because I lost all my trust in people. I was frightened to be hurt and I found I couldn't even look at people, which sounds like a really horrible thing to say, but I just couldn't. I just seemed to lose all emotions apart from anger, resentment and hatred, so although I still looked after my family in a practical way I think the deep love I used to feel for them just went, I just lost that, and it has been one of the hardest things for me to realise that I have to make a conscious effort to see the good in people and not just always be looking with suspicion for the bad in them.

I used to trust everybody, I used to think the world was a safe place but gradually I became paranoid. I took every little bit of trivia someone said to me very personally because I was already doubting my self-worth because of finding myself powerless over alcohol. So I began to feel powerless over other things in my life. I just bite and overreact to everything. I think I can learn in here how to react differently and how to accept that other people are just human as well, they have rotten days, so I needn't take everything so much to heart. I am trying to look at my positives now because beforehand I never took the time to look at my good points.

I think during the early years with him, my own self-esteem was at a fairly high level I didn't notice any difference in it but with the benefit of hindsight I can now see his alcohol problem was chipping away at me ever so slowly. I just didn't notice the negative build-up it was having on me. However, looking back now I think on some level I must have been aware things were going wrong because I spent an arm and a leg on confidence building work-shops and self-help books, all about assertiveness training, confidence building, having successful relationships with men and the like—none of which worked can I say—but I suppose they did distract my attention from him for a while. Although they brought about no lasting changes in me at all.

You know it is very difficult to live with someone who is always emotionally volatile and not very often on an even keel and if I get sucked into that it is not good for me. I think I got into the habit of putting up with a lot of unreasonable behaviour just to avoid the conflict that inevitably broke out when I tried to stand my ground. At the bottom of him I think he was at war within himself. Then when the kids arrived we had more responsibilities and I didn't know then that alcoholics tend to drink more at those times to escape the added responsibilities of life. I have only recently learned that in here from other people's experiences but at the time I had no idea why he had started to retreat from me and the kids. I thought it must have been something I'd done wrong so I think I must have unconsciously developed a sense of guilt about it and was forever trying to do better and try harder but it was all futile, nothing worked long-term.

I can also see now that I'd become very isolated because we had stopped going out and mixing with people. We would go to parties and he would end up with his head in the punch bowl. Well that can only happen a certain amount of times before you just become so embarrassed and not only do you stop accepting invites but other people stopped inviting us, so that affected my self-esteem as well.

Gradually I started to feel all these negative emotions and my resentment tipped over so it was greater than the good opinion I had once had of him. My anger tipped over too, so it was bigger than the joy I had, until finally I became this miserable git as well. He was always a lot more miserable than me but it was almost as if I was being sucked down into this pit of despair he was already in. Yet, I still had the arrogance to think I was the one who could save him and I bloody well couldn't! What really happened was he pulled me in with him and I couldn't get out either.

So when I arrived in AL I was in a heap and the realisation has started to dawn on me about the kind of life I have been living and I'm getting really angry with myself. I've started asking myself—What was I doing? What was I putting the kids through?"

Ingrid becomes too upset to speak and rummages through her bag for a packet of tissues before continuing.

"But I didn't see it at the time because I had no understanding of how alcoholism affected not only the drinker but our whole family.

I think when our self-esteem is knocked to such an extent by living with alcoholism it isn't just the relationship with the alcoholic that suffers. It's when we go out into the world and have any contact with anybody because our behaviour is affected by the way we are feeling as a result of what we have got to deal with at home.

So I would go out and I would have all of this anxiety and all of this worry and all of this exhaustion and then I would be meeting up for coffee with somebody and I would be going in like a wet rag and needless to say it didn't go terribly well. So then I come away thinking oh well there's another relationship that's not going well and that knocks my self-esteem again and before I know where I am my whole world was wrong and it just effected everything I did. So every time I was knocked that would be another reason why I would shrink, it's like a loop I got into that I just couldn't get out of.

I suppose I am just a common sense type of person and that approach had worked for me in my life. I had a very successful academic career and felt very confident at work. Up until then my world had been ruled by common sense, and I had always succeeded with that, but alcoholism would not be subjected to common sense. It was beyond reason and I had no idea how to conquer it. Still I thought I could because I had always been able to solve other things in my life.

Since coming to AL I have learned from listening to recovering alcoholics share that it is not the drinking, it's the thinking that causes the problem. Alcoholics seem to have a different pattern of thinking. So I was dealing with someone whose thinking was so very different to mine. Our realities were different and my life just turned into this big pan of spaghetti I couldn't untangle. I just kept thinking well what can I do to sort out this mess but I had no solutions. And I honestly believe if I hadn't found my way to AL and learned about this programme I would have had very little hope of ever finding my way back from the brink.

I don't know whether I will ever get me back to the giggly person I once was, but one of my greatest pleasures was getting up on a dance floor and dancing and I have started to do that again in the last couple of weeks. I can forget about everything while I'm dancing. Slowly I'm getting my self-esteem back to do that.

When I first met my husband I think I kind of sensed that he was wearing a mask and underneath he was sort of lonely and me in my wisdom thought I am the girl to cheer him up. But I didn't realise what I was taking on because I had never experienced that depth of despair and misery that he seems to have, so I couldn't know what I was taking on."

She pauses.

"And I think I'll just leave it there, Fadia. Thank You."

<u>GROUP TOGETHER</u>

"Thanks Ingrid."

<u>VICKY</u>

"I will come in Fadia, thanks Ingrid for your share and thanks everybody for being here."

Vicky is a relatively recent member of AL but she has spent a couple of years chaperoning her daughter to AA meetings. She is desperate to gain as much knowledge from others as she can in as short a space of time as possible.

"I think everyone who has the problem of alcoholism in their lives cannot get away without their self-esteem being knocked and mine was really low. Our daughter blamed us, and in particular me, for her alcoholism. I felt in a very fragile state at that time because I was living and breathing alcoholism 24hrs a day and all the other problems that go with it, it was just horrendous at the time. When we were able to catch her sober and ask her why she drank to excess it was always to do with us and the way she was brought up, the fact she was an only child and she didn't want to go to this school and basically blaming us for the alcoholism. Then there were other people who found out about this problem and said well why does she drink, what's the cause of this drinking? And we knew what they were thinking, they thought we were to blame too. So it was very hard and we were really on the bottom at that time. I started to get paranoid.

The one thing that kept me going was my job I used to look forward to going to work because I had to concentrate on my job and I could push the problem to the back of my mind for a while. I was quite good at my job, conscientious and I got on with people so I felt as if I was a better person at work. But then I would come home again and these horrible thoughts would come back and it took quite a long time in AL before I could believe I had any good points. I do like to help people if I can and it makes me feel better to help others so maybe that is a way I have of boosting my self-esteem. But alcoholism certainly knocked my confidence for six and I still feel I have a long way to go but I am better than I was."

GROUP TOGETHER

"Thanks Vicky."

FADIA

"I think I'll just say a few words here.

I was so full of resentment and emotional pain when I came here that I was poisoning myself with negativity without knowing it. My healing started with Step 4. I've now been able to forgive a lot of things and put them behind me. I started by writing letters to my grandmother—and not posting them—because she was the one I most resented, not my drunken grandfather. I feel I grew up being very repressed because she had always told me I had to keep my mouth shut with outsiders and not to tell anyone what went on inside our house.

I became very good at keeping secrets and this kept me distanced from everyone. I lived in constant fear that other people would find out about how we lived and would look down on us so I never felt good enough and had very little self-esteem. Of course what my grandmother was really teaching me was not to trust anyone. When I read the letters back I could see a lot of myself in them. I was repeating a lot of my grandmother's negative habits and it opened the door to some painful memories for me. Although it made me feel worse for a while it did teach me a lot more about myself and how my own behaviour patterns were self-sabotaging and stopping me from making a success of my own life. I have worked on Step 4 a lot because there was just so much baggage to deal with but I have found out so much about myself that I didn't know before, so it's been well worth my efforts.

I thought after Step 4, all the other steps would be easy. But No, in fact, I found Step 5 just as tough to do because I had such a fear of my imperfections that I didn't want to reveal them to anyone. But all of that has changed now and I love being imperfect today, it is such a relief."

GROUP TOGETHER

"Thanks Fadia."

JEFF

"I will come in Fadia."

Jeff is married to Alice. They usually come to the meetings together, although Alice is not at the meeting tonight. It is their son who is the alcoholic, who is still drinking and is drunk most days.

"It's not too difficult to understand really is it? That our self-esteem gets such a hammering. My story is much the same as others—one minute I was living in a nice world, with a nice house and a nice car and a lovely family and everything was going along great then out of the blue comes this alcoholism and it's just a big kick in the teeth. I tried to handle it, we tried to handle it like we had handled everything else in our married life, we just applied common sense really like Ingrid has already shared but it didn't work. I remember to the day—the feeling of devastation when this problem just wouldn't go away. What we had done all of our lives just wasn't working any more. It was frightening and then one thing leads to another and then we began to think—'well what have we done wrong? what caused this?' because we didn't know. Yes, we had many theories about what caused our son's alcoholism but the feeling that we could do absolutely nothing about it, it was then that I realised we had a weakness and this weakness just manifested itself all of the time.

Up until then I could do any job going, I would tackle anything but once this feeling of hopelessness with alcoholism came in, it took a very long time to try to pull things together again and get things back to normal.

I think the erosion of my self-esteem all started when I created this doubt in my own mind. We have all said it at some stage 'what have I done wrong?' That's the seed and I think we carry on from there and it just gets worse and worse. It's strange how I whipped myself. My main problem was I tried to deal with the alcohol situation the same way as I dealt with any other problem—with rationalisation, added to the fact that we all know better than the alcoholic. And that's being presumptuous really because the alcoholic has the right to do what they want to do whether I like it or not and whether it is good for them or not. It just made my self-esteem worse and worse because here was something I just couldn't solve, I didn't know how to deal with it and I had to learn it all in here. I also got the 'why me's?' and the 'what if's?' all sorted out in here.

I did all this with the support of the group. I have been coming here for a number of years and one of the big things that AL has taught me is not to always look at the dark side of life but to also look at the brighter things. And thanks to the support I've had I'm in a much better place now and I think Alice would say the same if she were here tonight.

Thank You."

GROUP TOGETHER

"Thanks Jeff."

STAVROS

"I would like to say just a few words Fadia."

The alcoholic in Stavros' life was his wife. He does not know whether she is still alive or not. The last time he heard any news of her, she was spotted living on the streets but he has never been able to track her down.

"Well it's a very hard thing to live with and I must admit it's done me the world of good coming here. I came into this meeting a long time ago, I make a joke of it today because there were 8 people all smiling and I hated every damned one of them because I was full of hell and I didn't really hear anything because my mind was back home wondering what my wife was doing. At that time I was focussing on everything except myself in my endeavour to stop her from drinking and it was detrimental to me both physically and mentally. It didn't do my children any good either because they saw me as the raving lunatic, disrupting the peace.

All the drunk wanted to do was go to sleep but I was waiting there behind the door whenever she came in, yelling "you're drunk again"!

However, what I did do from that very first meeting was I made myself a promise on the way home that I would go home and whatever happened when I got home I would stay quiet. It didn't matter what my wife said or did I would keep my mouth shut, which I did and it was a bit dramatic on that first occasion but slowly I got stronger in doing that. So instead of detaching through gritted teeth I started to do it with some feeling of compassion towards her and the day arrived when I found myself thinking poor soul. It was the understanding that alcoholism is a disease, an illness, and not a plot aimed at me. All the conflict that went on was simply

63

because she saw me as a threat to her drinking and her compulsion to drink was much greater than anything else in her life. She was a professional woman, a very well educated professional person, but that was irrelevant once the drink took hold. The drink became her first priority over everything else, including me and the kids.

My changed behaviour did not stop her drinking but it did change the entire atmosphere in the house and I didn't feel so uncomfortable about it in the end. I got a good night's sleep, I didn't jump out of bed every time I heard a car door slam or run to the window to see if it was her, or worry she might not even come home—and she would disappear for days on end when she was on a drinking bout.

When I first met her I knew something was wrong but I thought once we were married it would all be sorted, but five years later we were two lunatics in that house, it was a house of madness, her drunk and me trying to stop her drinking and nothing in the world was going to stop me from stopping her drinking.

When I came into AL I was told about changing my attitudes and I was absolutely furious. I didn't want to hear that. What me change? The cheeky so and so's I thought—why should I change? She was the lunatic not me. It was suggested I had to look to myself because there were things I could do to improve my situation. What I really needed was information about alcoholism and AL gave me that because people in this room understood where I was coming from.

Yes, I had already been to the doctors, already been to the psychiatrists, the clergy and whoever. They all nodded in the right places and invariably most of them said the wrong things—'chuck the bum out' and 'leave her' and all that rubbish. How was I going to do that when I loved this woman? I couldn't do that, so it was a change in my attitude which helped me to understand that here was a very intelligent, well-educated woman who was telling me she couldn't cope and I needed to learn to listen and to understand that. I'm not saying that this is what you must do, I am saying that that is what I had to do.

I told people in AL how I felt and they would tell me how they felt and I got the identification that I didn't get anywhere else. So, all the well-intended and well-meaning people who had studied their books couldn't help me because I needed someone who had lived with alcoholism to fully understand me. The so called helping professions can be sympathetic but I didn't want sympathy, I wanted empathy and for me it came from meetings like this.

Alcoholism is a terrible thing, it's not fun, no one comes in here skipping and singing. It's not like having a few drinks down the pub on a Saturday night with the rest of the crowd. My wife was just a slave to the bottle, once she started she couldn't stop. Besides the terrible financial problems and everyday chaos it caused, by far the worst thing for me was my own 'stinking thinking'—because when I put my whole focus on her and became obsessed with trying to stop her from drinking it just consumed my whole life and I was left just piling up heaps of anger and resentment all of which took years to undo further down the line in AL.

I lost contact with my friends, I stopped going out. At work I was just miles away because my head was in the clouds all the time and I just couldn't think properly. When I got home I didn't want to be there and I couldn't sleep properly. The first night I came here they told me I couldn't stop the drinking but she could, although that would have to be a decision she made for herself. Well that lifted a big weight off my shoulders. So instead of arguing and asking what she had been buying and looking in her bag for bottles, I just let her get on with it.

I still had the odd slip up now and again, because I am only human and there is only so much crap anyone can take, but I just had to learn to try and bite the bullet and keep quiet. I think it was the alcoholic's own frustration with her illness that triggered her aggressive outbursts at me. It wasn't really aimed at me because she was a different person when she was sober. It calmed me down a lot coming here and I know I want to keep coming back for as long as I feel I need help to recover from the impact this illness has had on me."

GROUP TOGETHER

"Thanks Stavros."

MACK

"I'll come in if I may Fadia."

Mack is a regular at AL meetings. He is a man of around 60 and comes from a family of Irish descent. He retired on grounds of ill-health at 52, which he believes is the result of obsessively trying to stop his alcoholic son from drinking.

"I see my self-esteem and self-worth as being like a rain-barrel which has to be constantly topped up or I am in big trouble. To top up my barrel I ask myself what talents have I got? What can I do? And I work with that information. I thought I was good at my job but eventually that came to nothing, probably because I was always being distracted by the chaos of alcoholism in the house.

However, I now seek out what I am good at and I think complements are great for topping up my barrel but the emptier my barrel becomes the more depressed, and even self-destructive, I can get. I constantly try to focus on my Step 4 talents and abilities and build on them. I leave working on my shortcomings for another day when I am feeling stronger. Over the years I had become disinterested in myself because I had spent all my time focusing on the alcoholic's antics and watching his every move. So in recovery I had to start asking myself what I could do Today to start developing my own abilities again. I did a Step 4 inventory of my talents and then asked myself what I would have to do to restart building up those talents again? The objective is to take charge of my own life even if it means taking risks and getting it wrong sometimes, at least, I'd be making my own choices and decisions about my own life again.

At first I couldn't even bring myself to look at Step 4, it was just too frightening. I wanted to put it away in a drawer and not look at it. Now I can't for the life of me see why I was so frightened because when I did finally get around to doing it, it was OK really. This shows me the strength I have been able to build up in my self-esteem because the time did come when I was not fearful at all to look at it."

<u>GROUP TOGETHER</u>

"Thanks Mack."

<u>PIPPA</u>

"I will just briefly come in Fadia."

Pippa attended a few AL meetings last year but decided it wasn't for her. She came back last week because she has recently left her alcoholic boyfriend and is sleeping on a friend's sofa. She feels at this time she needs the support of the group.

"Can I just say I have been practising 'detachment with compassion' all week and it is really helping me. My partner has been ringing and leaving messages blaming me for everything that's gone wrong in our relationship and he says if I just change everything would be OK with us. Which is just so not true but his angry tone sends me back to being a jittering child who is about to be crushed, I have such a fear of arousing other people's anger and will do anything to prevent it, so I am really glad to be here tonight in this safe place.

I know I need to develop some coping devices to deal with this rather than just avoiding it. I suppose I need to learn how to fight really. I'm sick of taking all his criticisms and just salving my wounds with excuses for his crap behaviour. I need to learn to set limits on what I'm prepared to accept from him but I have no confidence in my own judgement at the moment. Anyway, I've felt a bit calmer today, so thank you everybody."

<u>GROUP TOGETHER</u>

"Thanks Pippa."

CLARISSA

"I'll come in Fadia."

Clarissa is women in her mid 30's with 3 young children and an alcoholic husband who was in AA for 2 years, but has recently picked up again. She is hoping he decides to go back to AA again but she knows that has to be his decision.

"Well we all know there are some horrific effects of alcoholism but for me I think this is one of the worst because I think it is so tragic that alcoholism robs a lot of us of our self-esteem and you know we sit here week after week and we know how wonderful certain people are and yet we have so little opinions of ourselves. For me, I think there is also a combination of a childhood thing, my mum died when I was 10 and there were three of us kids. My dad was quite a domineering man and we were all afraid of him. I ended up leaving home at 16 to make a life for myself but then living for so many years with alcoholism I don't think I realised just how much it had destroyed my self-esteem.

Like other members have already shared tonight, I have been living this almost schizophrenic life where on the one hand, I have been doing a job where I was well respected and I knew I was pretty good at what I did, yet at other times not having any confidence over silly little things. And one of the struggles for me is, I know. I can see what alcoholism has done to me and a lot of other people and this problem of self-esteem is huge but I'm not sure how we regain our self-esteem. I think most of us still in some way blame ourselves for particular situations. But the other thought when I think of self-worth and self-esteem is—and this might sound a bit crazy, but children who witness domestic violence suffer terribly from low self-esteem and often they are never able to regain that in their lives and I wonder sometimes if I am a bit like that? Having lived with alcoholism for so many years that on one level I know I am good at certain things and I help people if I can and I've got lots of friends, I make an effort with my friends, I'm reliable and yet there is still this habit of being hard on myself.

In fact I am mostly very hard on myself and that is a pattern of mine which I have found very difficult to change. I think a lot of my own self-esteem has been thwarted because of my perfectionism. I thought I had to be super-woman and never ask for help from anyone or it was a sign of weakness but I see all that for the tosh it is now. Today I love being imperfect. It's such a relief. I now feel as if I tried to fix my husband mainly to save myself from having these uneasy emotions to deal with myself. I painted over the cracks really to keep myself happy. I wanted my life to run smoothly and he was blocking that. Which is OK, but at least I can be honest with myself now as to my true motives and not just think it is all the alcoholics doing.

I was a kind of robot really. Not thinking for myself and at everyone's beck and call. People just had to click their fingers and I would be there. I was always confident in my practical skills because I had practised them so much I was good at them. However, I can see now that I had very little self-esteem at all.

In my childhood my father demanded obedience, he didn't want us kids to love him he just wanted us to obey him. Being the only girl I think my role in the family was to take care of others needs and not to expect anything for myself. So now I have a very hard time knowing what I need or want or what my talents are. My childhood was a barrage of criticisms about my competence from my father so I think I had started out with a fairly low self-esteem and therefore any criticism from the alcoholic sparked off these painful childhood memories, which makes me want to try even harder and double my efforts to please. But as we find out in here, that is not the solution to the alcoholic's problem, in fact, it is just enabling him. I think I was frightened into abandoning any aspirations I ever had to keep in line with my father's demands. My saving grace has been my job, I have always loved my job teaching primary school children. Any self-esteem I have ever built up in my own life has been centred on my job. That is the only area where I have felt I have been able to live my own life and do my own stuff.

But it makes me feel really sad, this problem of self-esteem because although it was a hard road to come here and a hard reason why I came, the people I have met in AL are diamonds and I just wish I could wave a magic wand for everyone in here to show them just how good they are."

GROUP TOGETHER

"Thanks Clarissa."

Fadia keeps an eye on the time.

FADIA

"Well we have a few minutes left of the meeting if anyone would like to come in with a short share?"

JOSH

"I will come in Fadia.

This is my third meeting and I am amazed at the shares I hear in this room. Everyone is just so honest and I feel it is so uplifting and heart-warming to hear other people have come through this and are finding happiness and manageability in their lives again. I have taken on board the suggestion of putting my focus on my own life and doing my own stuff. This change in perspective has given me hope that maybe things can get better for me in time.

Thank you."

GROUP TOGETHER

"Thanks Josh."

FADIA

"Can I just remind our recent members we suggest you come back for at least 6 meetings before you decide whether it's for you or not. The reason we say that is because we have different members and different topics here at different times and it could be that you don't find anyone you feel you can identify with at your first few meetings. However, if after 6 meetings you find no identification then the group is probably either not for you or not for you at this time.

Before we close our meeting tonight I will just remind everybody of the theme for next time which will be—**Courage**

Do we have a volunteer to be the main sharer for next time?"

There is a pause.

EDDIE

"I will be the main sharer Fadia."

FADIA

"Thank You Eddie.

So it just remains for me to say that there are no dues for membership but we do ask you to make a contribution of whatever you can afford to cover our costs for tea and coffee and rent. If you cannot afford anything then that is OK too.

OK, I'm afraid our time is up and we close on time.

So Eddie, can I ask you to read the suggested closing to close our meeting please?"

EDDIE

"In closing, I would like to say that the opinions expressed here were strictly those of the person who gave them. Take what you liked and leave the rest. A few words to those of you who haven't been with us long: whatever your problems, there are those amongst us who have had them too. If you try to keep an open mind, you will find help.

You will come to realise that there is no situation too difficult to be bettered and no unhappiness too great to be lessened.

Will all those who care to, join me in closing our meeting?"

Everyone joins hands in a circle.

<u>GROUP TOGETHER</u>

"Grant me the Serenity to accept the things I cannot change.

The courage to change the things I can and

The wisdom to know the difference.

Same time, Same Place, Keep coming back, it works if you work it."